Keto Crock Pot Cookbook #2020

5-Ingredient Affordable, Easy & Delicious Keto Crock Pot Recipes | Lose Weight, Balance Hormones & Reverse Diabetes | 30-Day Keto Meal Plan

Dr Julane Soudel

Table of contents

Introduction

Struggling to lose weight? Suffering constantly from various ailments?

Obviously, your problems have something to do with your diet.

The link between food and health has long been established in scientific research.

In fact, a primary component of a healthy lifestyle is a healthy diet.

If you do not adopt a healthy diet, it's likely that you will suffer from excessive weight and all sorts of health problems, including but not limited to hypertension, diabetes, heart disease and so on.

One of the most popular diets that actually started many decades ago is the ketogenic diet.

If you do a quick research about it, you will find out that more and more people are turning to this diet program as a means to drop unwanted pounds as well as a way to improve overall health.

In this eBook, we will not only discuss about ketogenic diet, we will also provide delicious and easy-to-prepare ketogenic recipes prepared using the crockpot, one of the most reliable, efficient and versatile cooking appliances that can help you save both time and effort inside the kitchen.

Find out today how you can start your journey to a healthier lifestyle using this cookbook containing keto recipes using the crockpot.

Cheers!

Chapter 1: Why Keto Diet?

What is the Keto Diet?

Most people make the mistake of thinking that the ketogenic diet is the same as Atkins and other low-carb diet programs.

Yes, the keto diet also requires significant reduction in carbohydrate intake, but that's not all.

Aside from dramatically reducing your intake of carbs, it also replaces this with fat. It also requires moderate intake of protein.

Simply put, the keto diet is a low-carb, high-fat and moderate-protein diet program that you can adopt to lose weight and improve health.

It comes in several types, which include:

- Standard Ketogenic Diet – This keto diet program requires intake of 75% fat, 20% protein and 5% carbohydrates.
- Cyclical Keto Diet – With this particular keto diet, you will have to undergo phases of higher intake of carbohydrates. For example, you will go through 5 days of low-carb intake to be followed by two or three days of high-carb intake.
- Targeted Ketogenic Diet – This is the type of keto diet that enables you to put in more carbs during exercise periods.
- High Protein Ketogenic Diet – In this keto diet, you will include more protein and less fat. The portions include 60% fat, 35% protein and 5% carbs.

In this book, we will focus primarily on the first type of keto diet, the standard ketogenic diet that is most commonly used by people who aim to lose weight and improve health. The other types are more commonly used by weight trainers, bodybuilders and athletes.

Now, it probably makes you wonder how one can lose weight taking in more fat. We will discuss the amazing process by how this diet program works in the next section.

How Does the Ketogenic Diet Work?

The main method by which the keto diet works is this: you reduce your intake of carbs and increase fat. At the same time, you ensure that you take in moderate protein.

Doing this puts your body in a state referred to as ketosis.

As you know, the body makes use of carbs for energy. Meanwhile, fat is stored in the body for backup, and is what causes you to gain weight.

In the absence or lack of carbs, the body is forced to make use of the fat stored in your body, or the fat that you take in, and convert it into energy. This results in weight loss, more energy and better health.

The process inevitably lowers the levels of blood sugar and insulin, and this brings in numerous benefits for the health.

How to Know When You are in Ketosis

To determine if you have already reached the state of ketosis, here are some of the signs that you should watch out for. Some of these are positive while some are not so pleasant. But don't worry, once your body adopts to the change in your diet, the unpleasant signs will eventually go away on their own.

- Bad breath – Many keto dieters report that they suffer from having bad breath after reaching the state of ketosis. This is actually a common effect not only of the keto diet but also other low carb diets. This is caused by the increase in the levels of ketones in the blood, particularly acetone, which is emitted through breath and urine. It would be a good idea to brush your teeth many times during the day or chew on sugar-free gum.

- Weight loss – The main purpose of the ketogenic diet is to help you lose weight. Once you notice that you've been dropping significant amount of weight, then it's a good sign that you have reached the state of ketosis. Quick weight loss usually occurs in the first week. After that, you will lose weight more steadily.

- Increased blood ketones – There is also a significant reduction in the levels of blood sugar and a steady increase in the ketones. The most effective way to measure ketones is using the blood ketone meter, which calculates the number of beta-hydroxybutyrate in your blood. Ketosis has occurred when the blood ketones range from 0.5 to 3 mmol/L.

- Suppressed appetite – Many people who undergo this type of diet also relate that they experience the feeling of fullness, and that it now takes them a longer time to get hungry. The reason behind this has not yet been established in scientific research.

- Increased energy and better concentration – It's also common for keto dieters to experience a spike in energy, to feel less lethargic even during busy days, and to get better focus at work. Scientists have long investigated about how ketones are an effective source of fuel for the brain, helping in memory, focus and overall brain function.

- Digestive problems – This one is a side effect not only in ketogenic diet but in any other diet program. When the body shifts into a new diet, the digestive system is the first to take the hit. Adjusting to a new diet program usually results in digestive issues such as diarrhea or constipation. But these problems go away without any treatment a few days or weeks after you start the new diet.

The Health Benefits of Keto diet

There are many benefits to the ketogenic diet. These include the following:

- Reduces the appetite – It's true that hunger is the number one hindrance to weight loss diets. This is one of the best benefits that you'll get from the keto diet. When you start this diet, you will notice that you will feel full longer, and you will have fewer hunger pangs, which make it easier for you to lose weight.
- Helps you lose weight – Of course, this is a benefit that we cannot ignore. After all, this is the reason why most people adopt this diet. The ketogenic diet has been proven in various studies to be a highly effective means of losing weight not only for short-term but for long-term. In one study, it was found that the ketogenic diet is more effective than convention weight loss diet plans.
- Helps you cut down belly fat – The fat under your belly tend to make it difficult for your internal organs to work properly. You will find the fat loss in the abdominal cavity that you'll experience from keto diet truly beneficial for your overall health.
- Increases good cholesterol and reduces bad cholesterol – The ketogenic diet has been proven effective in increasing levels of high-density lipoprotein (HDL), more commonly known as the good cholesterol while at the same time, reducing the levels of low-density lipoprotein (LDL). This results in a significant reduction in heart disease risk.
- Reduces blood sugar levels – This is a benefit that people suffering from diabetes love about the ketogenic diet. Studies show that diabetic patients that adopt the ketogenic diet are able to drop insulin dosage by up to 50 percent.

8 Helpful Tips for the Keto Journey

Here are some practical tips that will help you on your journey with the ketogenic diet:

- Don't force yourself to eat three meals a day – Since there are times that you will feel full, you may not want to eat three full meals during the day, and this is perfectly fine. If you want to eat only twice a day, that is acceptable especially during the first few weeks.

- Focus more on healthy fats – Some people make the mistake of thinking that just because the keto diet is high in fat, you are forced to eat whatever type of fat you can get your hands on. While it's okay to eat bacon every now and then, you should still make an effort to focus more on healthy fats such as olive oil, avocado oil, nuts, fatty fish, avocado and so on.
- Don't forget about protein intake – Keep in mind that the keto diet is not just a high fat and low carb diet, you also need to have moderate intake of protein for it to work efficiently.
- Don't be too hard on yourself – Starting a new diet, whatever it is, can be difficult, stressful and daunting. Take it easy. Do not punish yourself if you fail a few times at first. You will eventually get the hang of things. Just be patient.
- Make dishes ahead – This is how the slow cooker helps. By using the crockpot, it becomes easier to plan and make your dishes ahead so you don't get tempted to rail away from your diet.
- Keep it varied – Keep your dishes varied so you don't get bored with the diet. Don't feed yourself with chicken dishes all the time, or eat only vegetable dishes. Make it varied so you won't feel like dieting is a chore.
- Be aware of the risks – Like most other diet programs, the keto diet also comes with certain risks that you should be aware of such as the unpleasant side effects mentioned earlier.
- Consult your doctor first – Do not start this diet without first consulting your doctor. This diet is not suitable for pregnant and breastfeeding women, and for people who have certain medical conditions.

Chapter 2: The Basics of Crock Pot

How Does a Crock Pot Work?

The crockpot is a kitchen appliance that is a type of a slow cooker.
A slow cooker is designed to create meals by slowly cooking the ingredients over either low or high heat.
It works by trapping the heat inside the device and cooking food for a much longer period. This brings out the flavor of the food, and simmers ingredients in their own juice for long hours. This creates rich and deep flavors that you can't get from grilling, frying and baking.

The Benefits of a Crock Pot

The crockpot is easy to use and economical. It saves you time, energy and even money.
It saves time and effort because it requires minimal active preparation on your part. You simply have to dump the ingredients in the crockpot, and set it to do its job. You can leave it and attend to other important tasks on hand.
It also helps save money because it allows you to make use of cheaper cuts of meat. Slow cooking cheaper cuts results in tender and succulent meat that you can't get by just frying or boiling.

Tips and Tricks for Using a Crock Pot

Here are some helpful tips and tricks for using your crockpot:

- Read the manual – Just like when you're using a new appliance for the first time, it's imperative that you first read the manual of your crockpot to ensure that you know how it works, and you know how to take good care of it. Most have two settings: low setting which cooks food between six and 10 hours, and high setting, which cooks food between four and six hours.
- Do not leave your home or sleep while cooking – While you can leave the crockpot to do its job of cooking your food, it is still not advisable to leave it alone in the house or to sleep and leave it on cooking overnight.
- Use liners to make cleaning easier – There are liners that you can use inside the crockpot so that it'll be easier and quicker for you to clean it up.
- Thaw frozen meat or poultry first before cooking – This quickens the cooking process and ensures that the food is cooked evenly.
- Do not overcrowd your crockpot – Make sure that you don't fill up your crockpot to the brim and to leave some space for heat to circulate.

Chapter 3: Foods to eat

Here's a quick list of food that you can eat while you're on a keto diet:

- Meat - Steak, ham, sausage, bacon, pork, lamb, beef
- Poultry – Chicken, turkey, duck
- Fatty fish – Salmon, tuna, mackerel, trout
- Cheese – Cheddar, goat cheese, cream cheese, blue cheese, mozzarella, Parmesan cheese
- Nuts and seeds – Almonds, flax seeds, walnuts, peanuts, pumpkin seeds, chia seeds
- Low-carb vegetables – Leafy greens, onions, bell peppers, green beans, tomatoes
- Healthy oils – Olive oil, avocado oil, coconut oil
- Condiments – Salt, pepper, herbs, spices
- Avocado
- Eggs
- Butter

Chapter 4: Foods to avoid

For the list of foods to avoid, here are those that you should watch out for. Just take note that some of these can be consumed but only in limited amount.

- Sugary beverages – Fruit juices, soda
- Sugary foods – Cakes, ice cream, candies, pastries, cookies
- Grains and starches – Rice, pasta, cereals
- Fruits – Most fruits except berries
- Root vegetables – Potatoes, sweet potatoes, carrots
- Sugary condiments and sauces
- Alcohol

Chapter 5: 30-Day Meal plan

Day 1

Breakfast: Bacon, Egg & Kale Casserole

Lunch: Zucchini Lasagna

Dinner: Meatballs

Day 2

Breakfast: Breakfast Sausage

Lunch: Shrimp Boil

Dinner: Balsamic Chicken

Day 3

Breakfast: Garlic Sausage with Egg & Broccoli Bake

Lunch: Stuffed Taco Peppers

Dinner: Beef Curry

Day 4

Breakfast: Sweet Potato Breakfast Casserole

Lunch: Ranch Chicken

Dinner: Salmon with Lemon & Dill

Day 5

Breakfast: Breakfast Casserole

Lunch: Beef Pot Roast

Dinner: Stewed Veggies

Day 6

Breakfast: Bacon, Egg & Kale Casserole

Lunch: Lamb Shanks with Green Beans

Dinner: Sesame Ginger Chicken

Day 7

Breakfast: Sausage & Broccoli Breakfast Casserole

Lunch: Zucchini Lasagna

Dinner: Shrimp Scampi

Day 8

Breakfast: Bacon & Egg Breakfast

Lunch: Cauliflower Pizza

Dinner: Salmon with Lemon & Dill

Day 9

Breakfast: Breakfast Bake

Lunch: Mongolian Beef

Dinner: Sesame Ginger Chicken

Day 10

Breakfast: Cauliflower Hash Browns

Lunch: Lamb with Thyme

Dinner: Salmon with Lemon Cream Sauce

Day 11

Breakfast: Breakfast Casserole

Lunch: Shrimp Jambalaya

Dinner: Beef & Broccoli

Day 12

Breakfast: Breakfast Sausage

Lunch: Fish Stew

Dinner: Balsamic Chicken

Day 13

Breakfast: Spicy Breakfast Casserole

Lunch: Barbecue Pulled Pork

Dinner: Tikka Masala

Day 14

Breakfast: Breakfast Bake

Lunch: Squash & Zucchini

Dinner: Meatballs

Day 15

Breakfast: Sausage & Broccoli Breakfast Casserole

Lunch: Vegetarian Curry

Dinner: Crack Chicken

Day 16

Breakfast: Eggs, Leeks & Mushrooms

Lunch: Beef Stroganoff

Dinner: Shrimp Scampi

Day 17

Breakfast: Breakfast Frittata

Lunch: Salmon with Lemon Cream Sauce

Dinner: Chicken with Green Beans

Day 18

Breakfast: Breakfast Casserole

Lunch: Tuscan Garlic Chicken

Dinner: Pork Curry

Day 19

Breakfast: Bacon & Egg Breakfast

Lunch: Stewed Veggies

Dinner: Greek Chicken

Day 20

Breakfast: Breakfast Bake

Lunch: Beef Stroganoff

Dinner: Cheesy Broccoli Quiche

Day 21

Breakfast: Sausage & Broccoli Breakfast Casserole

Lunch: Chicken Fajitas

Dinner: Spicy Pork Chops

Day 22

Breakfast: Cauliflower Hash Browns

Lunch: Fish Stew

Dinner: Lamb Shanks with Green Beans

Day 23

Breakfast: Breakfast Sausage

Lunch: Carnitas

Dinner: Seafood Bisque

Day 24

Breakfast: Ham & Egg Casserole

Lunch: Stuffed Taco Peppers

Dinner: Shrimp & Sausage Gumbo

Day 25

Breakfast: Eggs, Leeks & Mushrooms

Lunch: Pork Roast with Creamy Gravy

Dinner: Greek Chicken

Day 26

Breakfast: Bacon & Egg Breakfast

Lunch: Tikka Masala

Dinner: Cauliflower Pizza

Day 27

Breakfast: Hash Brown & Turkey Bacon

Casserole

Lunch: Crack Chicken

Dinner: Pulled Pork

Day 28

Breakfast: Egg, Tomato, Basil and Goat Cheese Omelet.

Lunch: Beef Curry

Dinner: Salmon with Lemon & Dill

Day 29

Breakfast: Breakfast Frittata

Lunch: Greek Chicken

Dinner: Vegetarian Curry

Day 30

Breakfast: Eggs, Leeks & Mushrooms

Lunch: Salmon with Lemon Cream Sauce

Dinner: Beef & Broccoli

Chapter 6: Breakfast and Brunch

Breakfast Bake

Preparation Time: 15 minutes
Cooking Time: 2 hours
Servings: 12

Ingredients:

- 10 strips bacon
- ½ cup onion, chopped
- ½ cup sweet red pepper, chopped
- 2 lb. ground sausage
- 12 eggs
- ½ cup heavy cream
- Salt and pepper to taste
- 4 cups cheddar cheese

Method:

1. In a pan over medium heat, cook the bacon until golden and crispy.
2. Chop into bits and then set aside.
3. Add the onion and red peppers to the pan.
4. Cook for 3 minutes.
5. Add the sausage and cook until brown.
6. Beat the eggs in a bowl.
7. Add the heavy cream to the eggs and season with salt and pepper.
8. Add the sausage mixture to your slow cooker.
9. Sprinkle cheese and bacon on top of the sausage mixture.
10. Pour egg mixture on the topmost layer.
11. Cover the pot and cook on high for 2 hours.

Nutritional Value:

- Calories 518
- Total Fat 40 g
- Saturated Fat 12 g
- Cholesterol 25 mg
- Sodium 250 mg
- Potassium 550 mg

- Total Carbohydrate 2 g
- Dietary Fiber 0 g
- Protein 34 g
- Total Sugars 3 g

Breakfast Casserole

Preparation Time: 10 minutes
Cooking Time: 7 hours
Servings: 8

Ingredients:

- 12 eggs
- ¾ cup milk
- Salt to taste
- ¾ teaspoon ground paprika
- 1 tsp. dried oregano
- Cooking spray
- 2 ½ cups cauliflower, blanched
- 1 red bell pepper, chopped
- 1 lb. sausage slices, cooked
- 1 ½ cup cheddar cheese, grated

Method:

1. Combine the eggs and milk.
2. Season with the salt, paprika and oregano.
3. Spray the bottom of the pot with oil.
4. Alternate the layers of the ingredients with the cauliflowers at the bottom most of the pot topped with the red bell pepper, sausage and cheese.
5. Pour the egg mixture on top most layer.
6. Cover the pot and cook on low for 7 hours.

Nutritional Value:

- Calories 379
- Total Fat 29 g
- Saturated Fat 11 g
- Cholesterol 310 mg
- Sodium 606 mg
- Potassium 418 mg
- Total Carbohydrate 4 g
- Dietary Fiber 0 g
- Protein 23 g
- Total Sugars X g

Bacon, Egg & Kale Casserole

Preparation Time: 15 minutes
Cooking Time: 1 hour and 40 minutes
Servings: 4

Ingredients:

- 3 bacon slices
- 3 tablespoons shallots, chopped
- 1 cup mushrooms, chopped
- ½ cup red bell pepper, chopped
- 9 leaves kale, shredded
- 6 eggs
- Salt and pepper to taste
- 1 tablespoon butter
- 1 cup Parmesan cheese, grated

Method:

1. Cook bacon in a pan until golden and crispy.
2. Add the shallots, mushrooms and red bell pepper.
3. Sauté for 1 to 2 minutes.
4. Stir in the kale and remove from heat.
5. In a bowl, mix the eggs, salt and pepper.
6. Put your slow cooker over high heat and put the butter inside.
7. Once the butter has melted, add the vegetables.
8. Pour the egg mixture into the pot.
9. Sprinkle with the cheese on top.
10. Cook on high for 1 hour and 30 minutes.

Nutritional Value:

- Calories 313
- Total Fat 22.2 g
- Saturated Fat 9.8 g
- Cholesterol 200 mg
- Sodium 826 mg
- Potassium 503 mg
- Total Carbohydrate 4 g
- Dietary Fiber 2.1 g
- Protein 22.9 g
- Total Sugars 3 g

Breakfast Sausage

Preparation Time: 10 minutes
Cooking Time: 3 hours and 10 minutes
Servings: 6

Ingredients:

- 1 lb. pork sausage
- 1 teaspoon dried sage
- 1 teaspoon dried thyme
- ½ teaspoon garlic powder
- Salt and pepper to taste
- ½ cup red bell pepper, chopped
- ½ cup green bell pepper, chopped
- ½ cup onion, chopped
- 1 tablespoon ghee
- 12 eggs
- ½ cup coconut milk
- 1 tablespoon nutritional yeast

Method:

1. Put a skillet over medium heat.
2. Let it heat for 2 minutes.
3. Cook the pork sausage for 3 minutes, breaking it into small pieces.
4. Season with the dried herbs, spices, salt and pepper.
5. Cook for another 5 minutes.
6. Add the bell peppers and onion.
7. Brush the pot with the ghee and pour in the pork and veggie mixture.
8. In a bowl, mix the rest of the ingredients.
9. Pour the mixture into the pot.
10. Cover the pot.
11. Cook on low for 3 hours.

Nutritional Value:

- Calories 461
- Total Fat 37.2g
- Saturated Fat 15.2g
- Cholesterol 396mg

- Sodium 694mg
- Potassium 471mg
- Total Carbohydrate 4.6g

- Dietary Fiber 1.3g
- Protein 27.3g
- Total Sugars 2.3g

Sausage & Broccoli Breakfast Casserole

Preparation Time: 10 minutes
Cooking Time: 3 hours
Servings: 8

Ingredients:

- Cooking spray
- 1 broccoli, chopped
- 12 oz. sausage links, cooked and sliced
- 1 cup cheddar cheese, shredded
- 10 eggs
- 2 cloves garlic, crushed and minced
- ¾ cup whipping cream
- Salt and pepper to taste

Method:

1. Spray the bottom part of your slow cooker.
2. Arrange layers of half of the following: broccoli, sausage and cheese.
3. Repeat the layers.
4. In a bowl, combine the rest of the ingredients.
5. Pour the egg mixture over the layers.
6. Cover the pot.
7. Cook on high for 3 hours.

Nutritional Value:

- Calories 484
- Total Fat 38.8 g
- Saturated Fat 16.5 g
- Cholesterol 399 mg
- Sodium 858 mg
- Potassium 675 mg
- Total Carbohydrate 5.39 g
- Dietary Fiber 1.18 g
- Protein 26.1 g
- Total Sugars 5 g

Ham & Egg Casserole

Preparation Time: 10 minutes
Cooking Time: 1 hour and 30 minutes
Servings: 4

Ingredients:

- Cooking spray
- 1 tablespoon butter
- 1 lb. ham, sliced into cubes
- 2 stalks green onion, chopped
- 6 eggs
- ½ cup heavy cream
- 1 cup cheese, shredded
- Salt and pepper to taste

Method:

1. Spray the bottom of the slow cooker with oil.
2. Add the butter.
3. Stir in the green onions and ham.
4. In a bowl, beat the eggs and mix with the cream.
5. Pour the egg mixture over the ham and green onions.
6. Sprinkle cheese on top.
7. Season with salt and pepper.
8. Cook on high for 1 hour.
9. Stir and cook on high for an additional 30 minutes.

Nutritional Value:

- Calories 446
- Total Fat 31 g
- Saturated Fat 16 g
- Cholesterol 367 mg
- Sodium 1745 mg
- Potassium 519 mg
- Total Carbohydrate 2.5 g
- Dietary Fiber 0 g
- Protein 37 g
- Total Sugars 2 g

Cauliflower Hash Browns

Preparation Time: 15 minutes
Cooking Time: 6 hours
Servings: 10

Ingredients:

- Cooking spray
- 12 eggs
- ½ cup milk
- Salt and pepper to taste
- ½ teaspoon dry mustard
- 1 head cauliflower, shredded
- 1 onion, diced
- 10 oz. precooked breakfast turkey sausage
- 2 cups cheddar cheese, shredded

Method:

1. Spray your slow cooker with oil.
2. Beat the eggs in a bowl.
3. Stir in the milk, salt, pepper and dry mustard.
4. Put 1/3 of the cauliflower in the bottom of the slow cooker.
5. Top with the 1/3 of the onion, 1/3 of the sausage and 1/3 of the cheese.
6. Repeat layers twice with the remaining ingredients.
7. Pour the egg and milk mixture over the layers.
8. Cook on low for 6 hours.

Nutritional Value:

- Calories 111
- Total Fat 7g
- Saturated Fat 2.5g
- Cholesterol 203mg
- Sodium 128mg
- Potassium 307mg
- Total Carbohydrate 3.7g
- Dietary Fiber 0.9g
- Protein 9g
- Total Sugars 2.1g

Hash brown & Turkey Bacon Casserole

Preparation Time: 20 minutes
Cooking Time: 4 hours and 5 minutes
Servings: 8

Ingredients:

- Cooking spray
- 1 package frozen hash browns
- 12 slices turkey bacon
- 1 red bell pepper, diced
- 1 red bell pepper, diced
- 16 eggs
- Salt and pepper to taste
- 1 cup cheddar cheese, grated

Method:

1. In a pan over medium high heat, cook the turkey bacon until golden and crispy. Set aside.
2. Spray your slow cooker with oil.
3. Arrange in even layers the hash browns, bacon, onion and bell peppers.
4. In a bowl, beat the eggs and season with salt and pepper.
5. Pour the egg mixture over the layers.
6. Sprinkle the cheese on top.
7. Cook on high for 4 hours.

Nutritional Value:

- Calories 424
- Total Fat 24g
- Saturated Fat 7.2g
- Cholesterol 357mg
- Sodium 658mg
- Potassium 609mg
- Total Carbohydrate 9.4g
- Dietary Fiber 2.7g
- Protein 21.6g
- Total Sugars 2.7g

Bacon & Egg Breakfast

Preparation Time: 15 minutes
Cooking Time: 1 hour and 5 minutes
Servings: 8

Ingredients:

- 10 slices bacon, cooked and chopped
- 10 eggs, beaten
- 1 cup whipping cream
- 8 oz. cheddar
- Salt and pepper to taste
- 1 tablespoon butter
- 3 stalks green onion, chopped

Method:

1. Cook the bacon in a pan over medium heat.
2. Drain and chop the bacon.
3. In a bowl, beat the eggs and stir in the cream and cheese.
4. Season with salt and pepper.
5. Add the butter to the slow cooker.
6. Pour the egg mixture into the pot.
7. Sprinkle bacon on top.
8. Cover the pot.
9. Cook on high for 1 hour.
10. Sprinkle green onions on top before serving.

Nutritional Value:

- Calories 315
- Total Fat 23.5g
- Saturated Fat 10g
- Cholesterol 257mg
- Sodium 815mg
- Potassium 257mg
- Total Carbohydrate 2.2g
- Dietary Fiber 0.2g
- Protein 23.1g
- Total Sugars 0.7g

Sweet Potato Breakfast Casserole

Preparation Time: 20 minutes
Cooking Time: 8 hours and 10 minutes
Servings: 6

Ingredients:

- 1 tablespoon butter
- 4 sausage, crumbled
- 2 cups sweet potatoes, grated
- 1 onion, diced
- 2 garlic cloves, crushed and minced
- 8 mushrooms, sliced
- 1 red bell pepper, diced
- 12 eggs
- 1 cup coconut milk
- Salt and pepper to taste
- 1 green onion, sliced

Method:

1. Melt butter in a pan over medium heat.
2. Add onion and garlic. Cook for 2 minutes.
3. Add sausage and cook for 5 minutes.
4. Arrange sweet potato shreds on the bottom of the slow cooker.
5. Pour the onion and sausage mixture on top.
6. Arrange the mushrooms and bell pepper on top of the onion and sausage.
7. In a bowl, mix the eggs and coconut milk.
8. Stir in the salt and pepper.
9. Pour this mixture on top of the layers.
10. Cook on low for 8 hours.
11. Garnish with the green onion.

Nutritional Value:

- Calories 344
- Total Fat 22.9g
- Saturated Fat 13.2g
- Cholesterol 340mg
- Sodium 215mg
- Total Carbohydrate 11.4g

- Dietary Fiber 3.9g
- Total Sugars 4.5g
- Protein 15.7g
- Potassium 809mg

Breakfast Frittata

Preparation Time: 15 minutes
Cooking Time: 3 hours
Servings: 6

Ingredients:

- Cooking spray
- ¼ cup onion, diced
- 1 cup red bell pepper, diced
- ½ cup green bell pepper, diced
- ¾ cups spinach, chopped
- 8 eggs
- 1 ¼ cup sausage, cooked and crumbled
- Salt and pepper to taste

Method:

1. Spray your slow cooker with oil.
2. Combine all the ingredients and mix well.
3. Seal the pot.
4. Cook on low for 3 hours.
5. Slice and serve.

Nutritional Value:

- Calories 238
- Total Fat 16 g
- Saturated Fat 5 g
- Cholesterol 98 mg
- Sodium 844 mg
- Potassium 75 mg
- Total Carbohydrate 3 g
- Dietary Fiber 1 g
- Protein 20 g
- Total Sugars 2 g

Garlic Sausage with Egg & Broccoli Bake

Preparation Time: 15 minutes
Cooking Time: 2 hours and 5 minutes
Servings: 8

Ingredients:

- 6 cloves garlic, crushed and minced
- 1 lb. breakfast turkey sausage
- 3 cups broccoli florets, blanched
- 12 eggs
- ½ cup heavy cream
- 2 cups cheddar cheese
- 2 tablespoons fresh parsley, chopped
- Salt and pepper to taste

Method:

1. In a pan over medium heat, cook the garlic for 1 minute.
2. Add the sausage and cook for 10 minutes.
3. In your slow cooker, add the broccoli florets in the bottom most layer.
4. Add the sausage on top.
5. In a bowl, beat the eggs and stir in the rest of the ingredients.
6. Pour the egg mixture on top of the layers.
7. Cover the pot.
8. Cook on high for 2 hours.

Nutritional Value:

- Calories 250
- Total Fat 18.9g
- Saturated Fat 9.8g
- Cholesterol 286mg
- Sodium 285mg
- Potassium 260mg
- Total Carbohydrate 4.2g
- Dietary Fiber 1g
- Protein 16.7g
- Total Sugars 1.3g

Spicy Breakfast Casserole

Preparation Time: 15 minutes
Cooking Time: 3 hours
Servings: 12

Ingredients:

- Cooking spray
- 12 eggs
- 1 lb. sausage, cooked and crumbled
- 1 lb. bacon, cooked and chopped
- ½ cup milk
- 2 cups cheddar cheese, grated
- ½ white onion, diced
- 1 red bell pepper, diced
- 2 tablespoons hot sauce
- Salt and pepper to taste
- Chili pepper flakes

Method:

1. Spray your slow cooker with oil.
2. Beat the eggs in a large bowl.
3. Stir in the rest of the ingredients.
4. Cover the pot and cook on low for 3 hours.

Nutritional Value:

- Calories 425
- Total Fat 35 g
- Saturated Fat 13 g
- Cholesterol 236 mg
- Sodium 811 mg
- Potassium 298 mg
- Total Carbohydrate 3 g
- Dietary Fiber 2 g
- Protein 21 g
- Total Sugars 1 g

Breakfast Egg & Potato

Preparation Time: 15 minutes
Cooking Time: 2 hours
Servings: 12

Ingredients:

- 12 eggs
- ½ cup heavy cream
- ½ cup onion, chopped
- 4 cups cheddar cheese
- Salt and pepper to taste
- 3 cups potatoes, grated

Method:

1. Beat the eggs and cream in a bowl.
2. Stir in the onion and cheese.
3. Season with salt and pepper.
4. Arrange the potatoes on the bottom part of the slow cooker.
5. Pour the egg mixture over the potatoes.
6. Cover the pot.
7. Cook on low for 2 hours.

Nutritional Value:

- Calories 260
- Total Fat 18.7g
- Saturated Fat 10.5g
- Cholesterol 210mg
- Sodium 300mg
- Potassium 259mg
- Total Carbohydrate 7.3g
- Dietary Fiber 1g
- Protein 15.7g
- Total Sugars 1.2g

Chapter 7: Soups and Stews

Zucchini Soup

Preparation Time: 20 minutes
Cooking Time: 4 hours and 10 minutes
Servings: 6

Ingredients:

- Cooking spray
- 1 ½ lb. Italian sausage
- 2 cups celery, chopped
- 2 lb. zucchini, sliced
- 56 oz. canned diced tomatoes
- 1 red bell pepper, sliced
- 1 green bell pepper, sliced
- 1 cup onion, chopped
- Salt to taste
- 1 teaspoon white sugar
- 1 teaspoon dried oregano
- 1 teaspoon Italian seasoning
- 1 teaspoon dried basil
- ¼ teaspoon garlic powder
- 5 tablespoons Parmesan cheese, grated

Method:

1. Spray your pan with oil.
2. Cook the sausage until brown. Drain the fat.
3. Add the celery and cook for 10 minutes. Set aside.
4. Put the sausage mixture along with the rest of the ingredients except Parmesan cheese in your slow cooker.
5. Cover the pot.
6. Cook on low for 4 hours.
7. Sprinkle Parmesan cheese on top before serving.

Nutritional Value:

- Calories 389
- Total Fat 23.6 g
- Saturated Fat 8 g
- Cholesterol 49 mg
- Sodium 2218 mg

- Potassium 1359 mg
- Total Carbohydrate 25.8 g
- Dietary Fiber 6.3 g
- Protein 21.8 g
- Total Sugars 13 g

Chicken Taco Soup

Preparation Time: 15 minutes
Cooking Time: 7 hours
Servings: 8

Ingredients:

- 1 onion, chopped
- 15 oz. canned corn kernels
- 15 oz. canned black beans
- 16 oz. canned chili beans
- 10 oz. canned diced tomatoes
- 8 oz. tomato sauce
- 1 packet taco seasoning
- 3 chicken breast fillets
- 8 oz. cheddar cheese, shredded
- Crushed tortilla chips

Method:

1. Add all the ingredients except chicken breast, cheese and tortilla chips in your slow cooker.
2. Mix well.
3. Arrange the chicken breast fillets on top of the mixture.
4. Cover the pot.
5. Cook on low for 5 hours.
6. Take the chicken out of the pot and shred.
7. Put the shredded chicken back to the pot.
8. Cook on low for 2 hours.
9. Sprinkle cheese and garnish with tortilla chips before serving.

Nutritional Value:

- Calories 434
- Total Fat 17.7 g
- Saturated Fat 8 g
- Cholesterol 68 mg
- Sodium 1597 mg
- Potassium 550 mg
- Total Carbohydrate 12 g
- Dietary Fiber 5 g
- Protein 27.2 g
- Total Sugars 4 g

Broccoli & Cheese Soup

Preparation Time: 10 minutes
Cooking Time: 3 hours
Servings: 12

Ingredients:

- 2 cups water
- 2 cups chicken broth
- 2 tablespoons butter
- 8 oz. cream cheese
- 1 cup whipping cream
- ½ cup Parmesan cheese
- 5 cups broccoli florets
- 2 ½ cups cheddar cheese, shredded
- Salt and pepper to taste

Method:

1. Pour the water and broth into your slow cooker.
2. Stir in the butter, cream cheese and cream.
3. Add the Parmesan cheese and broccoli.
4. Cover the pot.
5. Cook on low for 3 hours.
6. Top with the cheddar and season with salt and pepper before serving.

Nutritional Value:

- Calories 230
- Total Fat 20g
- Saturated Fat 12.5g
- Cholesterol 63mg
- Sodium 370mg
- Potassium 210mg
- Total Carbohydrate 3.8g
- Dietary Fiber 1g
- Protein 9.8g
- Total Sugars 0.9g

Mexican Chicken Soup

Preparation Time: 15 minutes
Cooking Time: 4 hours
Servings: 5

Ingredients:

- 2 teaspoons oil
- 1 onion, chopped
- 1 tablespoon garlic, crushed and minced
- 4 chicken breast fillets
- 14 oz. canned roasted tomatoes
- 1 red bell pepper, chopped
- 1 ½ teaspoons cumin
- 1 teaspoon dried oregano
- 1 ½ teaspoon chipotle chili powder
- 1 ½ chicken stock
- 1 cup half and half
- ½ cup cream cheese
- 1 cup Mexican blend cheese
- Salt to taste
- Cilantro

Method:

1. Pour the oil into a pan over medium heat.
2. Add the onion and garlic. Cook for 2 minutes.
3. In the slow cooker, add the chicken breast fillet, tomatoes, onion, garlic, spices, chicken stock and salt.
4. Seal the pot.
5. Cook on high for 3 hours.
6. Add the rest of the ingredients except cilantro and cook on high for 20 minutes.
7. Take the chicken out and shred using 2 forks.
8. Put the shredded chicken back to the pot.
9. Garnish with cilantro before serving.

Nutritional Value:

- Calories 100
- Total Fat 25 g
- Saturated Fat 13 g
- Cholesterol 120 mg
- Sodium 446 mg

- Potassium 607 mg
- Total Carbohydrate 11 g
- Dietary Fiber 1 g
- Protein 28 g
- Total Sugars 4 g

Cheesy Cauliflower Soup

Preparation Time: 15 minutes
Cooking Time: 4 hours and 15 minutes
Servings: 8

Ingredients:

- 1 onion, chopped
- 6 cups cauliflower florets
- 2 cups water
- 1 cup chicken broth
- 2 cups almond milk
- 2 scoops protein bone broth flakes
- 1 teaspoon Dijon mustard
- 8 oz. cheddar cheese, shredded

Method:

1. Put the onion, cauliflower, water, broth, almond milk and bone broth flakes into your slow cooker.
2. Mix well.
3. Cover the pot.
4. Cook on low for 3 hours.
5. Transfer the contents to an immersion blender.
6. Pulse until smooth.
7. Put the mixture back to the pot.
8. Stir in mustard and cheese.
9. Cook until the cheese has melted.

Nutritional Value:

- Calories 158
- Total Fat 10 g
- Saturated Fat 7 g
- Cholesterol 29 mg
- Sodium 339 mg
- Potassium 291 mg
- Total Carbohydrate 5 g
- Dietary Fiber 1 g
- Protein 10 g
- Total Sugars 1 g

Beef & Vegetable Soup

Preparation Time: 25 minutes
Cooking Time: 6 hours and 10 minutes
Servings: 12

Ingredients:

- 1 teaspoon butter
- 2 lb. stew meat, cubed
- 2 tablespoons red wine vinegar
- 32 oz. reduced-sodium beef broth
- 1 onion, chopped
- ¼ cup green beans, sliced
- 6 oz. celeriac, diced
- ¼ cup carrot, diced
- 2 tablespoons tomato paste
- 28 oz. canned diced tomatoes
- 2 cloves garlic, crushed
- 1/2 teaspoon dried rosemary
- 1/2 teaspoon dried thyme
- Salt and pepper to taste
- 4 slices bacon, chopped and cooked

Method:

1. Add the butter to a pan over medium heat.
2. Cook the beef cubes until brown.
3. Season with salt and pepper. Set aside.
4. Reduce heat to medium low.
5. Transfer the liquid mixture to the slow cooker with the remaining broth.
6. Add the beef and the rest of the ingredients to the pot.
7. Mix well.
8. Cover the pot.
9. Cook on low for 6 hours.
10. Sprinkle bacon bits on top before serving.

Nutritional Value:

- Calories 212
- Total Fat 13 g
- Saturated Fat 7 g
- Cholesterol 200 mg
- Sodium 522 mg

- Potassium 750 mg
- Total Carbohydrate 6 g
- Dietary Fiber 1 g
- Protein 17 g
- Total Sugars 1 g

Taco Soup

Preparation Time: 15 minutes
Cooking Time: 4 hours
Servings: 8

Ingredients:

- 1 tablespoon butter
- 2 lb. ground beef
- 2 cloves garlic, crushed and minced
- ½ cup onion, diced
- 2 tablespoons homemade taco seasoning
- ½ teaspoon ancho chili powder
- 20 oz. canned Rotel with green peppers
- 8 oz. cream cheese
- ½ cup cilantro, chopped
- 4 cups beef broth

Method:

1. In a pan over medium heat, cook the onion and garlic for 2 minutes.
2. Add the ground beef and cook until brown.
3. Transfer the ground mixture to your slow cooker.
4. Stir in the rest of the ingredients.
5. Seal the pot.
6. Cook on low for 4 hours.

Nutritional Value:

- Calories 346
- Total Fat 19.1g
- Saturated Fat 10g
- Cholesterol 136mg
- Sodium 551mg
- Potassium 613mg
- Total Carbohydrate 2.2g
- Dietary Fiber 0.2g
- Protein 39.1g

Bacon & Chicken Chowder

Preparation Time: 30 minutes
Cooking Time: 7 hours and 15 minutes
Servings: 8

Ingredients:

- 4 tablespoons butter, divided
- 1 onion, sliced thinly
- 1 shallot, chopped
- 4 cloves garlic, crushed and minced
- 1 leek, trimmed and sliced
- 2 ribs celery, chopped
- 6 oz. mushrooms, sliced
- 2 cups chicken stock, divided
- 1 lb. chicken breasts
- 8 oz. cream cheese
- 1 cup heavy cream
- 1 lb. bacon, cooked crisp and crumbled
- Salt and pepper to taste
- 1 teaspoon garlic powder
- 1 teaspoon dried thyme

Method:

1. Add half of the butter to the slow cooker.
2. Add the onion, shallot, garlic, leek, mushroom and celery to the pot.
3. Pour in half of the stock.
4. Season with salt and pepper.
5. Cover the pot.
6. Cook on low for 1 hour.
7. While waiting, cook the chicken in butter in a pan over medium heat.
8. Cook until brown on both sides.
9. Slice into cubes and set aside.
10. Add the rest of the ingredients except the bacon to the pot.
11. Stir well.

12. Add the chicken cubes and bacon.
13. Cover the pot and cook on low for 6 hours.

Nutritional Value:

- Calories 355
- Total Fat 28 g
- Saturated Fat 13 g
- Cholesterol 101 mg
- Sodium 552 mg
- Potassium 670 mg
- Total Carbohydrate 6.4 g
- Dietary Fiber 2 g
- Protein 21 g
- Total Sugars 3 g

Buffalo Chicken Soup

Preparation Time: 10 minutes
Cooking Time: 4 hours and 10 minutes
Servings: 4

Ingredients:

- ½ tablespoon ghee
- ¼ cup onion, diced
- ¾ cup celery, sliced thinly
- 2 cups chicken broth
- ½ cup coconut milk
- ½ cup ranch dressing
- ¼ cup hot sauce
- Salt to taste
- ¼ teaspoon paprika
- ½ lb. chicken thighs
- 1 tablespoon tapioca starch
- Green onion, chopped

Method:

1. Add the ghee to a pan over medium heat.
2. Add the onion and celery.
3. Cook for 3 minutes.
4. Transfer to your slow cooker.
5. Add the rest of the ingredients except tapioca starch and green onion.
6. Stir well.
7. Cover the pot and cook on high for 3 hours.
8. In a bowl, mix the tapioca starch with 2 tablespoons cooking liquid.
9. Stir into the pot.
10. Cook for another 2 hours.
11. Shred the chicken and put it back to the pot.
12. Garnish with the green onions.

Nutritional Value:

- Calories 305
- Total Fat 26.2 g

- Saturated Fat 8.2 g
- Cholesterol 46 mg
- Sodium 933 mg
- Potassium 359 mg

- Total Carbohydrate 6.9 g
- Dietary Fiber 0.6 g
- Protein 11.9 g
- Total Sugars 1.1 g

Chapter 8: Vegetables and Vegetarian

Zucchini Lasagna

Preparation Time: 45 minutes
Cooking Time: 4 hours and 45 minutes
Servings: 8

Ingredients:

- 4 cups zucchinis, sliced into thin strips
- 1 tablespoon salt
- 2 tablespoons coconut oil
- 1 cup onion, diced
- 1 tablespoon garlic, minced
- ½ tablespoon ginger, minced
- 1 lb. ground turkey
- Pepper to taste
- 1 cup coconut milk
- ¼ cup low sodium soy sauce
- ¼ cup creamy peanut butter
- 1 tablespoon rice vinegar
- 2 tablespoons coconut sugar
- 2 tablespoons hot sauce
- 1 tablespoon fish sauce
- 1 tablespoon freshly squeezed lime juice
- 15 oz. ricotta cheese
- 1 egg
- ½ cup cilantro, chopped
- 2 cups Napa cabbage, chopped
- ½ cup water chestnuts, diced
- 8 oz. mozzarella cheese

Method:

1. Preheat your oven to 350 degrees F.
2. Arrange the zucchini slices in a baking pan.

3. Sprinkle salt on top.
4. Bake in the oven for 20 minutes.
5. While waiting, pour the coconut oil in a pan over medium heat.
6. Add the onion, garlic, ginger and turkey.
7. Season with pepper.
8. Cook for 10 minutes.
9. Stir in the coconut milk, soy sauce, peanut butter, vinegar, sugar, hot sauce, fish sauce and lime juice.
10. Bring to a boil and then simmer for 4 minutes.
11. Take the zucchini strips out of the oven and press with a paper towel to get rid of extra moisture.
12. In a bowl, beat the egg and cheese. Set aside.
13. Spray your slow cooker with oil.
14. Spread half of the turkey mixture on the bottom part.
15. Layer the zucchini on top of the turkey.
16. Top with the ricotta.
17. Sprinkle half of the cilantro, cabbage, water chestnuts and Mozzarella cheese.
18. Repeat the layers.
19. Cover the pot and cook on low for 4 hours.

Nutritional Value:

- Calories 444
- Total Fat 30.8g
- Saturated Fat 17g
- Cholesterol 110mg
- Sodium 1771mg
- Potassium 612mg
- Total Carbohydrate 12.1g
- Dietary Fiber 2.4g
- Protein 34.7g
- Total Sugars 4.1g

Stewed Veggies

Preparation Time: 20 minutes
Cooking Time: 4 hours and 16 minutes
Servings: 6

Ingredients:

- Olive oil
- 1 onion, chopped
- 1 red bell pepper, chopped
- 1 green bell pepper, chopped
- 2 cloves garlic, minced
- 2 cups vegetable broth
- 14 oz. canned diced tomatoes
- 15 oz. chickpeas, rinsed and drained
- 1 tablespoon curry powder
- 1 tablespoon maple syrup
- 1 tablespoon ginger, chopped
- Salt and pepper to taste
- 1 head cauliflower, sliced into florets
- 10 oz. baby spinach, chopped
- 1 cup coconut milk

Method:

1. Pour the oil into a pan over medium high heat.
2. Cook the onion and bell peppers for 5 minutes.
3. Add the garlic and cook for 1 minute.
4. Pour the mixture into your slow cooker.
5. Add the rest of the ingredients except the cauliflower, spinach and coconut milk.
6. Cover and cook on high for 3 hours.
7. Stir in the cauliflower. Cover and cook on high 1 hour.
8. Stir in the coconut milk and spinach. Cook on high for 10 minutes.

Nutritional Value:

- Calories 169
- Total Fat 10.6g

- Saturated Fat 8.7g
- Cholesterol 0mg
- Sodium 317mg
- Potassium 832mg
- Total Carbohydrate 16.2g
- Dietary Fiber 5g
- Protein 6g
- Total Sugars 8.4g

Cauliflower Pizza

Preparation Time: 15 minutes
Cooking Time: 3 hours
Servings: 4

Ingredients:

For the crust:

- 1 head cauliflower, chopped
- 2 eggs, beaten
- ½ cup Italian cheese blend, shredded
- 1 teaspoon dried Italian seasoning blend
- Salt to taste

For the toppings:

- ½ cup Alfredo sauce
- 1 ½ cups Italian cheese blend, shredded
- ½ teaspoon dried rosemary

Method:

1. Put the cauliflower in a food processor.
2. Pulse until consistency is similar to rice.
3. Transfer to a bowl and stir in the crust ingredients.
4. Spray oil on your slow cooker.
5. Press the mixture on the bottom part of the pot.
6. Spread Alfredo sauce on top.
7. Top with the cheese and rosemary.
8. Cover.
9. Cook on high for 3 hours.
10. Let sit for 30 minutes before slicing and serving.

Nutritional Value:

- Calories 275
- Total Fat 21 g
- Saturated Fat 5 g
- Cholesterol 113 mg
- Sodium 499 mg
- Potassium 110 mg

- Total Carbohydrate 4 g
- Dietary Fiber 2 g

- Protein 18 g
- Total Sugars 1 g

Squash & Zucchini

Preparation Time: 5 minutes
Cooking Time: 6 hours
Servings: 6

Ingredients:

- 2 cups zucchini, sliced
- 2 cups yellow squash, sliced
- ½ teaspoon salt
- ¼ teaspoon pepper
- 1 teaspoon garlic powder
- 1 teaspoon Italian seasoning
- ¼ cup butter, sliced into cubes
- ¼ cup Parmesan cheese, grated

Method:

1. Put zucchini and squash in a slow cooker.
2. Season with the salt, pepper, garlic powder and Italian seasoning.
3. Top with the butter and cheese.
4. Cover the pot.
5. Cook on low for 5 hours.

Nutritional Value:

- Calories 122
- Total Fat 9.9 g
- Saturated Fat 5 g
- Cholesterol 100 mg
- Sodium 369 mg
- Potassium 225 mg
- Total Carbohydrate 5.4 g
- Dietary Fiber 1.7 g
- Protein 4.2 g
- Total Sugars 3 g

Cheesy Broccoli Quiche

Preparation Time: 20 minutes
Cooking Time: 2 hours and 15 minutes
Servings: 8

Ingredients:

- Water
- 3 cups broccoli florets
- 9 eggs
- 8 oz. cream cheese
- ¼ teaspoon onion powder
- Salt and pepper to taste
- Cooking spray
- 2 cups cheddar cheese, divided

Method:

1. Fill your pot with water.
2. Place it over medium high heat and bring to a boil.
3. Once the water is boiling, add the broccoli florets.
4. Boil for 3 minutes.
5. Drain and rinse the broccoli under running water. Set aside.
6. In a bowl, beat the eggs and cream cheese.
7. Season with the onion powder, salt and pepper.
8. Spray your slow cooker with oil.
9. Arrange the broccoli in the bottom of the pot.
10. Sprinkle half of the cheddar cheese on top.
11. Pour the egg mixture on top.
12. Cover the pot.
13. Cook on high for 2 hours and 15 minutes.
14. Sprinkle remaining cheddar on top.
15. Let sit for 10 minutes before serving.

Nutritional Value:

- Calories 337
- Total Fat 27.6g
- Saturated Fat 15.6g
- Cholesterol 254mg

- Sodium 741mg
- Potassium 129mg
- Total Carbohydrate 4.6g

- Dietary Fiber 0g
- Protein 16.9g
- Total Sugars 1.4g

Stuffed Taco Peppers

Preparation Time: 15 minutes
Cooking Time: 4 hours
Servings: 6

Ingredients:

- 1 cup cauliflower rice
- 4 cups ground turkey
- 1 cup Monterey Jack cheese, shredded
- ½ teaspoon onion powder
- ½ teaspoon garlic powder
- 1 teaspoon chili powder
- 1 ½ tablespoons olive oil
- 6 red bell peppers, tops sliced off and seeded
- 1 cup water

Method:

1. In a large bowl, combine all the ingredients except the bell peppers and water.
2. Stuff each red bell pepper shell with the mixture.
3. Arrange these into your slow cooker.
4. Pour the water into your pot.
5. Cover the pot and cook on high for 4 hours.

Nutritional Value:

- Calories 250
- Total Fat 15.8 g
- Saturated Fat 7 g
- Cholesterol 107 mg
- Sodium 450 mg
- Potassium 760 mg
- Total Carbohydrate 4.02 g
- Dietary Fiber 3 g
- Protein 22.19 g
- Total Sugars 2 g

Tikka Masala

Preparation Time: 15 minutes
Cooking Time: 1 hour and 35 minutes
Servings: 5

Ingredients:

For the cauliflower:

- 1 head cauliflower, sliced into florets
- 1 tablespoon olive oil
- 1 teaspoon garam masala
- 1 teaspoon ground cumin
- ½ teaspoon cayenne pepper
- Salt to taste

For the sauce:

- 4 tablespoons butter
- 1 onion, diced
- 1 tablespoon ginger, minced
- 2 cloves garlic, minced
- 1 ½ teaspoon paprika
- 1 tablespoon garam masala
- ½ teaspoon cayenne pepper
- 1 ½ cups canned crushed tomatoes
- 1 teaspoon ground cumin
- ½ cup water
- ½ cup coconut cream
- Salt to taste
- ¼ cup cilantro, minced

Method:

1. Preheat your oven to 425 degrees F.
2. In a large bowl, toss the cauliflower florets in oil and spices under the cauliflower ingredients.
3. Put in a baking pan and bake for 30 minutes.

4. In your slow cooker over medium heat, melt the butter, and cook the onion, ginger and garlic for 5 minutes.
5. Stir in the rest of the ingredients except the cilantro.
6. Cover the pot and cook on high for 1 hour.
7. Garnish with the cilantro before serving.

Nutritional Value:

- Calories 248
- Total Fat 21.2 g
- Saturated Fat 10 g
- Cholesterol 37 mg
- Sodium 298 mg
- Potassium 716 mg
- Total Carbohydrate 4.5 g
- Dietary Fiber 3.6 g
- Protein 14.7 g
- Total Sugars 5.3 g

Vegetarian Curry

Preparation Time: 15 minutes
Cooking Time: 4 hours
Servings: 6

Ingredients:

- 3 cups coconut milk
- 2 tablespoons curry powder
- Salt to taste
- 1 teaspoon red pepper flakes, crushed
- 1 ½ teaspoons granulated garlic
- 6 cups pineapple chunks
- 1 lb. sweet potatoes, sliced
- 2 green bell peppers, sliced
- 2 onions, sliced

Method:

1. Combine all the ingredients in your slow cooker.
2. Mix well.
3. Cover the pot.
4. Cook on high for 4 hours.

Nutritional Value:

- Calories 291
- Total Fat 17.6g
- Saturated Fat 15.3g
- Cholesterol 0mg
- Sodium 34mg
- Potassium 772mg
- Total Carbohydrate 8g
- Dietary Fiber 6.1g
- Protein 3.6g
- Total Sugars 14.7g

Chapter 9: Poultry

Crack Chicken

Preparation Time: 15 minutes
Cooking Time: 4 hours
Servings: 8

Ingredients:

- ½ cup chicken broth
- 1 packet ranch seasoning
- 2 lb. chicken breast fillets
- 8 oz. cream cheese
- 8 slices bacon, cooked crispy and crumbled
- ½ cup cheddar cheese, shredded

Method:

1. Pour chicken broth into your slow cooker.
2. Add the ranch seasoning and chicken breast.
3. Stir well.
4. Cover the pot and cook on high for 4 hours.
5. Shred the chicken using two forks.
6. Put shredded chicken back to the pot.
7. Stir in the rest of the ingredients.
8. Cook for 10 more minutes.

Nutritional Value:

- Calories 347
- Total Fat 23 g
- Saturated Fat 10 g
- Cholesterol 125 mg
- Sodium 475 mg
- Potassium 520 mg
- Total Carbohydrate 1 g
- Dietary Fiber 2 g
- Protein 30 g
- Total Sugars 3 g

Chicken Fajitas

Preparation Time: 10 minutes
Cooking Time: 3 hours
Servings: 6

Ingredients:

- 1 ½ lb. chicken breast fillet
- ½ cup salsa
- 8 oz. cream cheese
- 1 teaspoon cumin
- 1 teaspoon paprika
- Salt and pepper to taste
- 1 onion, sliced
- 1 clove garlic, minced
- 1 red bell pepper, sliced
- 1 green bell pepper, sliced
- 1 teaspoon lime juice

Method:

1. Combine all the ingredients except the lime wedges in your slow cooker.
2. Cover the pot.
3. Cook on high for 3 hours.
4. Shred the chicken.
5. Drizzle with lime juice.
6. Serve with toppings like sour cream and cheese.

Nutritional Value:

- Calories 276
- Total Fat 17 g
- Saturated Fat 8 g
- Cholesterol 105 mg
- Sodium 827 mg
- Potassium 776 mg
- Total Carbohydrate 8 g
- Dietary Fiber 3 g
- Protein 25 g
- Total Sugars 2 g

Tuscan Garlic Chicken

Preparation Time: 15 minutes
Cooking Time: 3 hours
Servings: 6

Ingredients:

- 1 tablespoon olive oil
- 6 cloves garlic, crushed and minced
- ½ cup chicken broth
- 1 cup heavy cream
- ¾ cup Parmesan cheese, grated
- 4 chicken breasts
- 1 tablespoon Italian seasoning
- Salt and pepper to taste
- ½ cup sundried tomatoes, chopped
- 2 cups spinach, chopped

Method:

1. Pour the oil into your pan over medium heat.
2. Cook the garlic for 1 minute.
3. Stir in the broth and cream.
4. Simmer for 10 minutes.
5. Stir in the Parmesan cheese and remove from heat.
6. Put the chicken in your slow cooker.
7. Season with the salt, pepper and Italian seasoning.
8. Place the tomatoes on top of the chicken.
9. Pour the cream mixture on top of the chicken.
10. Cover the pot.
11. Cook on high for 3 hours.
12. Take the chicken out of the slow cooker and set aside.
13. Add the spinach and stir until wilted.
14. Pour the sauce over the chicken and serve with the sun-dried tomatoes and spinach.

Nutritional Value:

- Calories 306
- Total Fat 18.4g

- Saturated Fat 7.5g
- Cholesterol 115mg
- Sodium 287mg
- Potassium 482mg
- Total Carbohydrate 4.9g
- Dietary Fiber 0.8g
- Protein 30.1g
- Total Sugars 2g

Balsamic Chicken

Preparation Time: 15 minutes
Cooking Time: 4 hours
Servings: 8

Ingredients:

- 1 tablespoon olive oil
- 6 chicken breasts fillets
- 30 oz. canned diced tomatoes
- 1 onion, sliced thinly
- 4 cloves garlic
- ½ cup balsamic vinegar
- 1 teaspoon dried rosemary
- 1 teaspoon dried basil
- 1 teaspoon dried oregano
- ½ teaspoon thyme
- Salt and pepper to taste

Method:

1. Add the oil to your slow cooker.
2. Place the chicken breasts inside the pot.
3. Put the onions on top with the garlic cloves and herbs.
4. Pour the vinegar and tomatoes on top.
5. Cover the pot and cook on high for 4 hours.

Nutritional Value:

- Calories 238
- Total Fat 12 g
- Saturated Fat 3 g
- Cholesterol 73 mg
- Sodium 170 mg
- Potassium 550 mg
- Total Carbohydrate 7 g
- Dietary Fiber 2 g
- Protein 25 g
- Total Sugars 4 g

Sesame Ginger Chicken

Preparation Time: 5 minutes
Cooking Time: 5 hours
Servings: 4

Ingredients:

- 1 ½ lb. chicken breast fillet
- ½ cup tomato sauce
- ¼ cup low-sugar peach jam
- ¼ cup chicken broth
- 2 tablespoons coconut aminos
- 1 ½ tablespoons sesame oil
- 1 tablespoon honey
- 1 teaspoon ground ginger
- 2 cloves garlic, minced
- ¼ cup onion, minced
- ¼ teaspoon red pepper flakes, crushed
- 2 tablespoons red bell pepper, chopped
- 1 ½ tablespoons green onion, chopped
- 2 teaspoons sesame seeds

Method:

1. Combine all the ingredients except green onion and sesame seeds in your slow cooker.
2. Mix well.
3. Cover the pot and cook on high for 4 hours.
4. Garnish with the green onion and sesame seeds.

Nutritional Value:

- Calories 220
- Total Fat 13 g
- Saturated Fat 8 g
- Cholesterol 100 mg
- Sodium 246 mg
- Potassium 550 mg
- Total Carbohydrate 7 g
- Dietary Fiber 1 g
- Protein 26 g
- Total Sugars 2 g

Ranch Chicken

Preparation Time: 5 minutes
Cooking Time: 4 hours and 5 minutes
Servings: 6

Ingredients:

- 2 lb. chicken breast fillet
- 3 tablespoons butter
- 4 oz. cream cheese
- 3 tablespoons ranch dressing mix

Method:

1. Add the chicken to your slow cooker.
2. Place the butter and cream cheese on top of the chicken.
3. Sprinkle ranch dressing mix.
4. Seal the pot.
5. Cook on high for 4 hours.
6. Shred the chicken using forks and serve.

Nutritional Value:

- Calories 266
- Total Fat 12.9 g
- Saturated Fat 8 g
- Cholesterol 102 mg
- Sodium 167 mg
- Potassium 450 mg
- Total Carbohydrate 8 g
- Dietary Fiber 0 g
- Protein 33 g
- Total Sugars 3 g

Chicken with Green Beans

Preparation Time: 5 minutes
Cooking Time: 4 hours
Servings: 4

Ingredients:

- 1 onion, diced
- 2 cloves garlic, crushed and minced
- 2 tomatoes, diced
- ¼ cup dill, chopped
- 1 lb. green beans
- 1 cup chicken broth
- 1 tablespoon lemon juice
- 4 chicken thighs
- Salt and pepper to taste
- 2 tablespoons olive oil

Method:

1. Put the onion, garlic, tomatoes, dill and green beans in your slow cooker.
2. Pour in the chicken broth and lemon juice.
3. Season with salt and pepper.
4. Mix well.
5. Add the chicken on top of the vegetables.
6. Drizzle chicken with oil.
7. Cover the pot.
8. Cook on high for 4 hours.

Nutritional Value:

- Calories 373
- Total Fat 26 g
- Saturated Fat 6 g
- Cholesterol 111 mg
- Sodium 315 mg
- Potassium 726 mg
- Total Carbohydrate 14 g
- Dietary Fiber 4 g
- Protein 22 g
- Total Sugars 6 g

Greek Chicken

Preparation Time: 15 minutes
Cooking Time: 2 hours
Servings: 6

Ingredients:

- 2 tablespoons olive oil
- 3 cloves garlic
- 2 lb. chicken thigh fillets
- Salt and pepper to taste
- 1 cup kalamata olives
- 8 oz. marinated artichoke hearts, rinsed and drained
- 12 oz. roasted red peppers, drained and sliced
- 1 onion, sliced
- ½ cup chicken broth
- ¼ cup red wine vinegar
- 1 tablespoon lemon juice
- 1 teaspoon dried oregano
- 1 teaspoon dried thyme
- 2 tablespoons arrowroot starch

Method:

1. Season the chicken with salt and pepper.
2. Put a pan over medium high heat.
3. Add the oil and garlic.
4. Cook for 1 minute, stirring frequently.
5. Add the chicken and cook for 2 minutes per side.
6. Transfer the chicken to the slow cooker.
7. Add the olives, artichoke hearts and peppers around the chicken.
8. Sprinkle onion on top.
9. In a bowl, mix the rest of the ingredients except the arrowroot starch.
10. Pour this into the slow cooker.
11. Cover the pot.
12. Cook on high for 2 hours.
13. Get 3 tablespoons of the cooking liquid.

14. Stir in the arrowroot starch to the liquid and put it back to the pot.
15. Simmer for 15 minutes before serving.

Nutritional Value:

- Calories 452
- Total Fat 36 g
- Saturated Fat 9 g
- Cholesterol 159 mg
- Sodium 899 mg
- Potassium 366 mg
- Total Carbohydrate 4 g
- Dietary Fiber 1 g
- Protein 26 g
- Total Sugars 3 g

Chapter 10: Beef, Pork and Lamb

Beef Curry

Preparation Time: 10 minutes
Cooking Time: 8 hours and 10 minutes
Servings: 4

Ingredients:

- 250 ml coconut cream
- 1 teaspoon Chinese five spice
- 1 teaspoon turmeric
- ½ teaspoon chili powder
- 1 teaspoon ground cardamom
- 2 teaspoons ground coriander
- 4 cloves whole
- 1 teaspoon ground cinnamon
- 1 teaspoon ground cumin
- 1 onion, sliced into quarters
- 6 cups beef, sliced into thin strips
- 2 cups leafy greens

Method:

1. Add the coconut cream along with all the spices into your slow cooker.
2. Mix well.
3. Add the beef and onion.
4. Toss to coat evenly.
5. Cover the pot.
6. Cook on low for 8 hours.
7. Stir in the leafy greens 5 minutes before the cooking is done.

Nutritional Value:

- Calories 256
- Total Fat 14.1 g
- Saturated Fat 8 g
- Cholesterol 220 mg
- Sodium 350 mg
- Potassium 556 mg

- Total Carbohydrate 2 g
- Dietary Fiber 0.9 g
- Protein 29.1 g
- Total Sugars 1.4 g

Mongolian Beef

Preparation Time: 10 minutes
Cooking Time: 6 hours
Servings: 4

Ingredients:

- 1 ½ lb. sirloin steak, sliced
- ¼ cup sugar
- ¼ cup water
- ¼ cup soy sauce
- 2 cloves garlic, crushed and minced
- 2 tablespoons sesame oil
- ¼ teaspoon red pepper flakes
- ½ teaspoon ground ginger
- ¼ teaspoon xanthan gum
- 2 green onion, chopped

Method:

1. Add the beef to the slow cooker.
2. In a bowl, mix the brown sugar, water, soy sauce, garlic, oil, red pepper flakes and ginger.
3. Pour this mixture over the beef.
4. Cover the pot.
5. Cook on low for 6 hours.
6. Take out a tablespoon of the cooking liquid.
7. Add xanthan gum to the liquid.
8. Pour this mixture back to the pot.
9. Sprinkle green onion on top.

Nutritional Value:

- Calories 417
- Total Fat 25.4 g
- Saturated Fat 12 g
- Cholesterol 108 mg
- Sodium 257 mg
- Potassium 556 mg
- Total Carbohydrate 2 g
- Dietary Fiber 0.4 g
- Protein 35.7 g
- Total Sugars 2 g

Beef Stroganoff

Preparation Time: 15 minutes
Cooking Time: 6 hours
Servings: 4

Ingredients:

- 1 onion, sliced into wedges
- 2 cloves garlic, crushed
- 2 slices bacon, diced
- 1 lb. stewing steak, sliced into cubes
- 1 teaspoon smoked paprika
- 3 tablespoons tomato paste
- 250 ml. beef stock
- 1 cup mushrooms, sliced into quarters

Method:

1. Put all the ingredients in your slow cooker.
2. Mix well.
3. Cook on high for 6 hours.

Nutritional Value:

- Calories 317
- Total Fat 19 g
- Saturated Fat 9 g
- Cholesterol 105 mg
- Sodium 226 mg
- Potassium 557 mg
- Total Carbohydrate 8 g
- Dietary Fiber 1 g
- Protein 29 g
- Total Sugars 4 g

Beef Short Ribs

Preparation Time: 5 minutes
Cooking Time: 8 hours
Servings: 8

Ingredients:

- 1 tablespoon olive oil
- 2 lb. beef short ribs
- ½ cup beef broth
- 3 oz. cream cheese
- 1 teaspoon garlic powder
- 2 cups white mushrooms
- Salt and pepper to taste

Method:

1. Place the skillet in medium heat.
2. Add the oil and cook the ribs until brown.
3. Mix the rest of the ingredients in your slow cooker.
4. Seal the pot. Cook on low for 8 hours. Mix every 2 hours.

Nutritional Value:

- Calories 365
- Total Fat 33 g
- Saturated Fat 15 g
- Cholesterol 74 mg
- Sodium 422 mg
- Potassium 295 mg
- Total Carbohydrate 1 g
- Dietary Fiber 2 g
- Protein 13 g
- Total Sugars 3 g

Meatballs

Preparation Time: 10 minutes
Cooking Time: 4 hours
Servings: 8

Ingredients:

- Olive oil
- 1 lb. ground beef
- 1 lb. ground pork
- 1 egg
- ¼ cup mayonnaise
- ¼ cup pork rinds, crushed
- 2 tablespoons Parmesan cheese, grated
- Salt and pepper to taste

For the sauce

- 14 oz. chili sauce
- 12 oz. grape jam

Method:

1. Preheat your oven to 400.
2. Drizzle baking sheet with olive oil.
3. Combine the ground beef, pork, egg, mayo, pork rinds, cheese, salt and pepper.
4. Form into meatballs.
5. Bake in the oven for 15 minutes.
6. Add the sauce ingredients to the slow cooker.
7. Mix well.
8. Add the meatballs.
9. Cover the pot and cook on low for 8 hours.

Nutritional Value:

- Calories 263
- Total Fat 11.9g
- Saturated Fat 3.9g
- Cholesterol 120mg
- Sodium 203mg
- Potassium 475mg

- Total Carbohydrate 2.1g
- Dietary Fiber 0g
- Protein 35.3g
- Total Sugars 0.5g

Beef & Broccoli

Preparation Time: 10 minutes
Cooking Time: 6 hours
Servings: 2

Ingredients:

- 2/3 cup liquid amino
- 2 lb. flank steak, sliced into strips
- 3 tablespoons stevia
- 1 cup beef broth
- 3 cloves garlic, minced
- 1 teaspoon ginger, grated
- Salt to taste
- ½ teaspoon red pepper flakes
- 2 cups broccoli florets
- 1 red bell pepper, sliced into strips

Method:

1. Add all the ingredients except broccoli and red bell pepper into the slow cooker.
2. Seal the pot.
3. Cook low for 6 hours.
4. Stir in the broccoli and red bell pepper.
5. Cook for another 1 hour.

Nutritional Value:

- Calories 320
- Total Fat 13g
- Saturated Fat 5.3g
- Cholesterol 83mg
- Sodium 250mg
- Total Carbohydrate 4.5g
- Dietary Fiber 1.2g
- Total Sugars 1.7g
- Protein 44.1g
- Potassium 692mg

Beef Pot Roast

Preparation Time: 15 minutes
Cooking Time: 3 hours and 15 minutes
Servings: 10

Ingredients:

- 3 lb. chuck roast
- 1 teaspoon garlic powder
- Salt and pepper to taste
- ¼ cup balsamic vinegar
- 2 cups water
- ½ cup onion, chopped
- ¼ teaspoon xanthan gum
- Parsley, chopped

Method:

1. Sprinkle both sides of the chuck roast with garlic powder, salt and pepper.
2. In a pan over medium high heat, sear the roast until brown on both sides.
3. Pour the vinegar to deglaze the pan. Cook for 1 minute.
4. Transfer to your slow cooker.
5. Stir in the onion and water.
6. Boil and then cook on low for 3 hours.
7. Stir in the xanthan gum and simmer until sauce has thickened.
8. Garnish with parsley.

Nutritional Value:

- Calories 298
- Total Fat 11.3g
- Saturated Fat 4.1g
- Cholesterol 137mg
- Sodium 92mg
- Total Carbohydrate 0.8g
- Dietary Fiber 0.2g
- Total Sugars 0.3g
- Protein 45g
- Potassium 410mg

Carnitas

Preparation Time: 15 minutes
Cooking Time: 8 hours
Servings: 16

Ingredients:

- 2 tablespoons butter
- 1 onion, sliced
- 4 tablespoons garlic, minced
- 8 lb. pork butt, sliced with crisscross pattern on top
- 2 tablespoons cumin
- 2 tablespoons thyme
- 2 tablespoons chili powder
- Salt and pepper to taste
- 1 cup water

Method:

1. Add the butter to your slow cooker.
2. Arrange the onion and garlic on the bottom of the pot.
3. Rub the pork with the spices, salt and pepper.
4. Put the meat inside the pot.
5. Add the water.
6. Cover the pot.
7. Cook on high for 8 hours.
8. Shred the meat and serve.

Nutritional Value:

- Calories 609
- Total Fat 45 g
- Saturated Fat 20 g
- Cholesterol 120 mg
- Sodium 220 mg
- Potassium 540 mg
- Total Carbohydrate 5 g
- Dietary Fiber 1 g
- Protein 54 g
- Total Sugars 4 g

Pulled Pork

Preparation Time: 5 minutes
Cooking Time: 8 hours
Servings: 8

Ingredients:

- 3 lb. boneless pork shoulder
- 1 tablespoon parsley
- 2 teaspoons cumin
- 2 teaspoons garlic powder
- 2 teaspoons onion powder
- Salt to taste
- 2 teaspoons paprika
- ½ cup beer

Method:

1. Put the pork shoulder to your slow cooker.
2. In a bowl, mix all the spices and herbs with the salt.
3. Rub pork with this mixture.
4. Add beer to the slow cooker.
5. Cover your pot.
6. Cook on low for 8 hours.
7. Shred the meat with fork.
8. Serve warm.

Nutritional Value:

- Calories 511
- Total Fat 37 g
- Saturated Fat 13 g
- Cholesterol 153 mg
- Sodium 647 mg
- Potassium 570 mg
- Total Carbohydrate 2 g
- Dietary Fiber 0 g
- Protein 40 g
- Total Sugars 0 g

Pork Roast with Creamy Gravy

Preparation Time: 15 minutes
Cooking Time: 8 hours and 15 minutes
Servings: 6

Ingredients:

- 2 lb. pork shoulder
- Salt and pepper to taste
- 1 ½ cups heavy whipping cream
- 2 teaspoons dried rosemary
- 5 black peppercorns
- 1 bay leaf
- 1 cup water
- 1 tablespoon coconut oil
- 2 cloves garlic, chopped
- 1 ½ oz. fresh ginger, grated
- 1 tablespoon arrowroot starch

Method:

1. Season pork with salt and pepper.
2. Add to a slow cooker.
3. Pour in the water.
4. Add the rosemary, peppercorns and bay leaf.
5. Cover the pot.
6. Cook on low for 8 hours.
7. Take it out of the pot and transfer to a plate.
8. In a bowl, combine the oil, garlic and ginger.
9. Rub pork with this mixture.
10. Bake in the oven for 15 minutes.
11. Get the cooking liquid from the pot.
12. Mix with the arrowroot starch.
13. Slice the beef and pour gravy on top before serving.

Nutritional Value:

- Calories 592
- Total Fat 46.2g

- Saturated Fat 20.9g
- Cholesterol 177mg
- Sodium 118mg
- Potassium 624mg
- Total Carbohydrate 6.5g
- Dietary Fiber 1.1g
- Protein 36.6g
- Total Sugars 0.3g

Spicy Pork Chops

Preparation Time: 5 minutes
Cooking Time: 8 hours
Servings: 8

Ingredients:

- 1 tablespoon dried thyme
- 1 tablespoon dried rosemary
- 1 tablespoon chives, chopped
- 1 tablespoon curry powder
- 1 tablespoon ground cumin
- 1 tablespoon fennel seeds
- Salt to taste
- 4 tablespoons olive oil, divided
- 2 lb. pork chops

Method:

1. In a bowl, mix all the spices with salt and 1 tablespoon olive oil.
2. Rub pork chops with this mixture.
3. Place the meat to your slow cooker.
4. Pour in the remaining oil.
5. Cook on high for 8 hours.

Nutritional Value:

- Calories 247
- Total Fat 15 g
- Saturated Fat 3 g
- Cholesterol 75 mg
- Sodium 347 mg
- Potassium 466 mg
- Total Carbohydrate 1 g
- Dietary Fiber 1 g
- Protein 24 g
- Total Sugars 1 g

Pork Curry

Preparation Time: 10 minutes
Cooking Time: 10 hours
Servings: 10

Ingredients:

- 2 lb. pork belly
- 13 oz. coconut cream
- 14 oz. diced tomatoes
- ¼ teaspoon ground cloves
- ¼ teaspoon ground ginger
- ½ teaspoon granulated garlic
- 1 ½ teaspoon curry powder
- ½ teaspoon onion powder
- 2 teaspoons garam masala

For the dry rub:

- ½ teaspoon onion powder
- ½ teaspoon ground ginger
- ½ teaspoon ground cloves
- 1 tablespoon granulated garlic
- ½ teaspoon curry powder
- Salt and pepper to taste

Method:

1. Score the pork belly.
2. Mix all the dry rub ingredients in a bowl.
3. Season pork belly with this mixture.
4. Marinate in the refrigerator while covered for 2 hours.
5. In another bowl, mix the rest of the ingredients.
6. Pour the mixture into the slow cooker.
7. Add the pork belly.
8. Toss to coat evenly.
9. Cook on high for 10 hours, stirring occasionally.

Nutritional Value:

- Calories 616
- Total Fat 62 g
- Saturated Fat 29 g
- Cholesterol 65 mg
- Sodium 263 mg
- Potassium 386 mg
- Total Carbohydrate 5 g
- Dietary Fiber 1 g
- Protein 10 g
- Total Sugars 1 g

Barbecue Pulled Pork

Preparation Time: 15 minutes
Cooking Time: 6 hours
Servings: 6

Ingredients:

- ¼ cup white wine vinegar
- 2 teaspoons olive oil
- 3 teaspoons paprika
- 2 teaspoons dried oregano
- 2 teaspoons garlic powder
- Salt and pepper to taste
- ¾ teaspoons ground cumin
- 1 teaspoon chipotle powder
- ¼ teaspoon cayenne pepper
- 1 tablespoon erythritol
- 2 lb. pork shoulder, sliced into cubes
- 1 tablespoon olive oil
- 1 tablespoon orange juice
- 1 teaspoon arrowroot powder

Method:

1. Mix all the ingredients except orange juice and arrowroot powder.
2. Put the mixture into the slow cooker.
3. Cover the pot and cook on low for 6 hours.
4. Stir in orange juice and arrowroot powder.
5. Shred the meat and serve with the sauce.

Nutritional Value:

- Calories 294
- Total Fat 16 g
- Saturated Fat 4 g
- Cholesterol 102 mg
- Sodium 418 mg
- Potassium 587 mg
- Total Carbohydrate 3 g
- Dietary Fiber 1 g
- Protein 30 g
- Total Sugars 3 g

Lamb with Thyme

Preparation Time: 5 minutes
Cooking Time: 3 hours
Servings: 2

Ingredients:

- 2 lamb chops, trimmed
- 1 cup vegetable stock
- ½ cup red wine
- 1 teaspoon garlic paste
- ¼ cup fresh thyme
- Salt and pepper to taste

Method:

1. Add all the ingredients in your slow cooker. Mix well.
2. Cover and cook on high for 3 hours.
3. Pour sauce over the lamb before serving.

Nutritional Value:

- Calories 167
- Total Fat 20 g
- Saturated Fat 9 g
- Cholesterol 56 mg
- Sodium 474 mg
- Potassium 110 mg
- Total Carbohydrate 3 g
- Dietary Fiber 0.01 g
- Protein 56 g
- Total Sugars 1 g

Lamb Shanks with Green Beans

Preparation Time: 20 minutes
Cooking Time: 8 hours and 10 minutes
Servings: 6

Ingredients:

- 6 lamb shanks
- 1 tablespoon olive oil
- Salt and pepper to taste
- 2 carrots, chopped
- 2 stalks celery, chopped
- 1 onion, chopped
- 1 tablespoon dried oregano
- 1 cup red wine
- 1 ½ cups chicken stock
- 1 ½ tablespoons rosemary
- 1 cup crushed tomatoes
- 3 bay leaves
- 3 cups green beans, sliced
- 1 tablespoon olive oil

Method:

1. In a skillet, pour the oil and cook the lamb shanks until brown on all sides.
2. Transfer to a plate.
3. Add the vegetables and cook for 5 minutes.
4. Transfer to a slow cooker.
5. Pour the red wine into the pan to deglaze.
6. Transfer to the slow cooker.
7. Add all the spices, chicken stock and tomatoes to the pot.
8. Stir in the lamb shanks.
9. Cover the pot.
10. Cook on low for 8 hours.
11. Sauté the green beans in oil.
12. Serve the lamb shanks with the beans.

Nutritional Value:

- Calories 465
- Total Fat 23 g
- Saturated Fat 10 g
- Cholesterol 162 mg
- Sodium 162 mg

- Potassium 969 mg
- Total Carbohydrate 13 g
- Dietary Fiber 4 g
- Protein 43 g
- Total Sugars 4 g

Chapter 11: Seafood and Fish

Shrimp Scampi

Preparation Time: 15 minutes
Cooking Time: 3 hours
Servings: 4

Ingredients:

- ¼ cup chicken bone broth
- ½ cup white cooking wine
- 2 tablespoons olive oil
- 2 tablespoons butter
- 1 tablespoon garlic, minced
- 2 tablespoons parsley, chopped
- 1 tablespoon lemon juice
- Salt and pepper to taste
- 1 lb. shrimp, peeled and deveined

Method:

1. Mix all the ingredients in your slow cooker.
2. Cover the pot.
3. Cook on low for 3 hours.

Nutritional Value:

- Calories 256
- Total Fat 14.7 g
- Saturated Fat 8 g
- Cholesterol 23 mg
- Sodium 466 mg
- Potassium 475 mg
- Total Carbohydrate 2.1 g
- Dietary Fiber 0.1 g
- Protein 23.3 g
- Total Sugars 2 g

Shrimp Boil

Preparation Time: 15 minutes
Cooking Time: 4 hours
Servings: 4

Ingredients:

- 1 ½ lb. potatoes, sliced into wedges
- 6 cloves garlic, peeled
- 3 ears corn
- 1 lb. sausage, sliced
- ¼ cup Old Bay seasoning
- 1 tablespoon lemon juice
- 6 cups water
- 2 lb. shrimp, peeled

Method:

1. Put the potatoes in your slow cooker.
2. Add the garlic, corn and sausage in layers.
3. Season with the Old Bay seasoning.
4. Drizzle lemon juice on top.
5. Pour in the water.
6. Do not mix.
7. Cover the pot.
8. Cook on high for 4 hours.
9. Add the shrimp on top.
10. Cook for 15 minutes.

Nutritional Value:

- Calories 585
- Total Fat 25.1g
- Saturated Fat 7.9g
- Cholesterol 382mg
- Sodium 2242mg
- Potassium 1166mg
- Total Carbohydrate 35.7g
- Dietary Fiber 4.9g
- Protein 53.8g
- Total Sugars 3.9g

Shrimp Jambalaya

Preparation Time: 10 minutes
Cooking Time: 8 hours
Servings: 6

Ingredients:

- 1 lb. sausage, sliced
- 1 lb. chicken breast fillets, sliced into cubes
- 1 onion, chopped
- 1 cup celery, chopped
- 1 green pepper, chopped
- 28 oz. canned diced tomatoes
- 1 cup chicken broth
- 2 teaspoons parsley, chopped
- 2 teaspoons fresh oregano, chopped
- 1 teaspoon cayenne pepper
- 2 teaspoons Cajun seasoning
- 1 lb. shrimp, peeled
- ½ teaspoon fresh thyme, chopped
- Salt and pepper to taste

Method:

1. Put all the ingredients except the shrimp in a slow cooker.
2. Mix well.
3. Cook low for 8 hours.
4. Stir in the shrimp 30 minutes before cooking is done.

Nutritional Value:

- Calories 537
- Total Fat 29g
- Saturated Fat 9g
- Cholesterol 290mg
- Sodium 981mg
- Potassium 1005mg
- Total Carbohydrate 10.2g
- Dietary Fiber 2.9g
- Protein 56.4g
- Total Sugars 5.1g

Salmon with Lemon Cream Sauce

Preparation Time: 10 minutes
Cooking Time: 2 hours and 20 minutes
Servings: 6

Ingredients:

For the salmon

- 3 lemons, sliced and divided
- 2 lb. salmon fillet
- Cooking spray
- Salt and pepper to taste
- ½ teaspoon sweet paprika
- ½ teaspoon chili powder
- 1 teaspoon garlic powder
- 1 teaspoon Italian Seasoning
- 1 cup vegetable broth
- 1 tablespoon lemon juice

For the sauce

- 3 tablespoons lemon juice
- ¼ cup chicken broth
- 2/3 cup heavy cream
- Lemon zest

Method:

1. Cover slow cooker with parchment paper.
2. Arrange the lemon slices in the middle.
3. Put the salmon fillet on top.
4. Spray salmon with oil and season with herbs and spices.
5. Pour the lemon juice and broth into the slow cooker around and not on top of the fish.
6. Cover and cook on low for 2 hours.
7. Combine the sauce ingredients.
8. Stir into the pot.

9. Set it to low and cook for 8 minutes.
10. Garnish with the zest.

Nutritional Value:

- Calories 330
- Total Fat 19 g
- Saturated Fat 7 g
- Cholesterol 119 mg
- Sodium 240 mg
- Potassium 857 mg
- Total Carbohydrate 7 g
- Dietary Fiber 1 g
- Protein 31 g
- Total Sugars 1 g

Shrimp & Sausage Gumbo

Preparation Time: 15 minutes
Cooking Time: 1 hour and 15 minutes
Servings: 4

Ingredients:

- 3 tablespoons olive oil
- 2 lb. chicken thigh fillet, sliced into cubes
- 4 cloves garlic, crushed and minced
- 1 onion, sliced
- 3 stalks celery, chopped
- 1 green bell pepper, chopped
- 1 teaspoon Cajun seasoning
- Salt to taste
- 2 cups beef broth
- 28 oz. canned crushed tomatoes
- 12 oz. sausage
- 2 tablespoons butter
- 1 lb. shrimp, peeled and deveined

Method:

1. Pour the olive oil in a pan over medium heat.
2. Cook the garlic and chicken for 5 minutes.
3. Add the onion, celery and bell pepper.
4. Cook until tender.
5. Season with the Cajun seasoning and salt.
6. Cook for 2 minutes.
7. Stir in the sausage, broth and tomatoes.
8. Cover and cook on low for 1 hour.
9. Add the butter and shrimp in the last 10 minutes of cooking.

Nutritional Value:

- Calories 467
- Total Fat 33 g
- Saturated Fat 10 g
- Cholesterol 238 mg

- Sodium 1274 mg
- Potassium 658 mg
- Total Carbohydrate 8 g

- Dietary Fiber 2 g
- Protein 33 g
- Total Sugars 5 g

Fish Stew

Preparation Time: 15 minutes
Cooking Time: 1 hour and 24 minutes
Servings: 2

Ingredients:

- 1 lb. white fish
- 1 tablespoon lime juice
- 1 onion, sliced
- 2 cloves garlic, sliced
- 1 red pepper, sliced
- 1 jalapeno pepper, sliced
- 1 teaspoon paprika
- 2 cups chicken broth
- 2 cups tomatoes, chopped
- Salt and pepper to taste
- 15 oz. coconut milk

Method:

1. Marinate the fish in lime juice for 10 minutes.
2. Pour the olive oil into a pan over medium heat.
3. Add the onion, garlic and peppers.
4. Cook for 4 minutes.
5. Add the rest of the ingredients except the coconut milk.
6. Cover the pot.
7. Cook on low for 1 hour.
8. Stir in the coconut milk and simmer for 10 minutes.

Nutritional Value:

- Calories 323
- Total Fat 28.6g
- Saturated Fat 17.1g
- Cholesterol 0mg
- Sodium 490mg
- Potassium 487mg
- Total Carbohydrate 11.1g
- Protein 9.3g
- Dietary Fiber 3.2g
- Total Sugars 6.2g

Seafood Bisque

Preparation Time: 15 minutes
Cooking Time: 2 hours and 35 minutes
Servings: 4

Ingredients:

- 2 tablespoons coconut oil
- ¼ cup onion, diced
- 1 stalk celery, diced
- 1 leek, sliced
- 1 teaspoon orange zest
- 1 teaspoon fresh thyme
- 8 oz. cream cheese
- 3 cups chicken broth
- 2 tablespoons tomato paste
- Salt and pepper to taste
- 12 oz. shrimp, cooked

Method:

1. Add oil to a skillet over medium heat.
2. Cook the onion, celery, leek, orange zest and thyme for 4 minutes.
3. Transfer to a slow cooker.
4. Stir in the rest of the ingredients except the shrimp.
5. Cover the pot and cook on low for 2 hours.
6. Stir in the shrimp 30 minutes before cooking is done.

Nutritional Value:

- Calories 411
- Total Fat 29.2g
- Saturated Fat 19.1g
- Cholesterol 241mg
- Sodium 964mg
- Potassium 513mg
- Total Carbohydrate 9.3g
- Dietary Fiber 1.1g
- Protein 28.1g
- Total Sugars 2.8g

Salmon with Lemon & Dill

Preparation Time: 15 minutes
Cooking Time: 2 hours
Servings: 4

Ingredients:

- Cooking spray
- 1 teaspoon olive oil
- 2 lb. salmon
- 1 tablespoon fresh dill, chopped
- Salt and pepper to taste
- 1 clove garlic, minced
- 1 lemon, sliced

Method:

1. Spray your slow cooker with oil.
2. Brush both sides of salmon with olive oil.
3. Season the salmon with salt, pepper, dill and garlic.
4. Add to the slow cooker.
5. Put the lemon slices on top.
6. Cover the pot and cook on high for 2 hours.

Nutritional Value:

- Calories 313
- Total Fat 15.2g
- Saturated Fat 2.2g
- Cholesterol 100mg
- Sodium 102mg
- Potassium 900mg
- Total Carbohydrate 0.7g
- Dietary Fiber 0.1g
- Protein 44.2g
- Total Sugars 0g

Chapter 12: Desserts

Berry Mix

Preparation Time: 5 minutes
Cooking Time: 2 hours
Servings: 8

Ingredients:

- Cooking spray
- 2 cups frozen strawberries
- 2 cups frozen blackberries
- 2 cups frozen blueberries
- 1 tablespoon orange juice
- 1 teaspoon orange zest
- 2 tablespoons water

Method:

1. Spray your crockpot with oil.
2. Add all the ingredients in the pot.
3. Cover the pot.
4. Cook on low for 2 hours.

Nutritional Value:

- Calories 50
- Total Fat 0.3g
- Saturated Fat 0g
- Cholesterol 0mg
- Sodium 1mg
- Potassium 91mg
- Total Carbohydrate 12.2g
- Dietary Fiber 3.6g
- Protein 0.8g
- Total Sugars 7.8g

Winter Fruits

Preparation Time: 10 minutes
Cooking Time: 6 hours
Servings: 10

Ingredients:

- 1 cinnamon stick
- 2 apples, sliced
- ¼ cup dried cranberries
- ¼ cup raisins
- ½ cup dried apricots
- 8 oz. pineapple chunks
- ¾ cup orange juice

Method:

1. Add all the ingredients in your crockpot.
2. Seal the pot.
3. Cook on low setting for 6 hours.
4. Discard cinnamon stick before serving.

Nutritional Value:

- Calories 59
- Total Fat 0.2g
- Saturated Fat 0g
- Cholesterol 0mg
- Sodium 1mg
- Potassium 162mg
- Total Carbohydrate 15g
- Dietary Fiber 1.8g
- Protein 0.6g
- Total Sugars 11.4g

Peach & Blackberry

Preparation Time: 20 minutes
Cooking Time: 3 hours
Servings: 12

Ingredients:

- 1 cup rolled oats
- 2 teaspoons ground cinnamon
- 1 teaspoon ground nutmeg
- ½ cup butter
- Cooking spray
- 3 lb. peaches, sliced
- 3 cups blackberries
- Walnuts, chopped

Method:

1. Combine all the ingredients except walnuts in a bowl.
2. Transfer to your crockpot.
3. Spray your pot with oil.
4. Cover and cook on low for 3 hours.
5. Sprinkle walnuts on top.

Nutritional Value:

- Calories 217
- Total Fat 9.2 g
- Saturated Fat 5 g
- Cholesterol 20 mg
- Sodium 101 mg
- Potassium 650 mg
- Total Carbohydrate 8 g
- Dietary Fiber 3 g
- Protein 25 g
- Total Sugars 5 g

Spiced Peaches

Preparation Time: 10 minutes
Cooking Time: 4 hours
Servings: 6

Ingredients:

- Cooking spray
- 4 cups frozen peaches, sliced
- 1 teaspoon ground cinnamon
- ½ teaspoon ground nutmeg
- 1 teaspoon vanilla extract
- ½ cup almond milk

Method:

1. Spray your slow cooker with oil.
2. In a bowl, mix all the ingredients.
3. Transfer to the pot.
4. Cover and cook on low for 3 hours.

Nutritional Value:

- Calories 287
- Total Fat 27 g
- Saturated Fat 12 g
- Cholesterol 30 mg
- Sodium 397 mg
- Potassium 295 mg
- Total Carbohydrate 7 g
- Dietary Fiber 5 g
- Protein 14 g
- Total Sugars 4 g

Cinnamon Strawberries

Preparation Time: 5 minutes
Cooking Time: 1 hour
Servings: 4

Ingredients:

- 4 cups frozen strawberries
- 2 tablespoons ground cinnamon
- 1 tablespoon ground nutmeg
- 1 cup orange juice
- Flaxseed

Method:

1. Mix all the ingredients except flaxseed in your crockpot.
2. Seal the pot and cook on low for 1 hour.
3. Sprinkle flaxseed on top before serving.

Nutritional Value:

- Calories 96
- Total Fat 0.8g
- Saturated Fat 0.5g
- Cholesterol 0mg
- Sodium 1mg
- Potassium 145mg
- Total Carbohydrate 8 g
- Dietary Fiber 5.3g
- Protein 0.7g
- Total Sugars 14.7g

Fruit Salad

Preparation Time: 10 minutes
Cooking Time: 2 hours
Servings: 10

Ingredients:

- ¾ cup sugar
- ½ cup butter
- ¼ teaspoon ground cinnamon
- ¼ teaspoon ground nutmeg
- Salt to taste
- 15 oz. peaches, sliced
- ½ cup dried apricots
- ½ cup dried blackberries
- Chopped walnuts

Method:

1. Combine all the ingredients except the walnuts in the crockpot.
2. Mix well.
3. Seal the pot and cook on high for 2 hours.
4. Sprinkle with the walnuts before serving.

Nutritional Value:

- Calories 326
- Total Fat 19 g
- Saturated Fat 8 g
- Cholesterol 24 mg
- Sodium 115 mg
- Potassium 445 mg
- Total Carbohydrate 6 g
- Dietary Fiber 3 g
- Protein 10 g
- Total Sugars 6 g

Fruit Medley

Preparation Time: 10 minutes
Cooking Time: 1 hour
Servings: 8

Ingredients:

- 1 cup frozen cherries
- 1 cup dried cranberries
- 1 cup frozen strawberries
- 1 cup frozen blueberries
- 1 teaspoon vanilla extract
- 1 teaspoon cinnamon
- 1 cup butter
- ¼ cup chopped almonds

Method:

1. Put all the ingredients except the almonds in the crockpot.
2. Seal the pot and cook on high for 1 hour.
3. Sprinkle almonds on top before serving.

Nutritional Value:

- Calories 256
- Total Fat 24.7g
- Saturated Fat 14.7g
- Cholesterol 61mg
- Sodium 164mg
- Total Carbohydrate 8.6g
- Dietary Fiber 2.2g
- Total Sugars 5.4g
- Protein 11.2g
- Potassium 92mg

Fruit Crisp

Preparation Time: 4 hours
Cooking Time: 15 minutes
Servings: 6

Ingredients:

- 6 cups apples, sliced
- 1 cup dried cranberries
- 1 teaspoon orange zest
- 5 teaspoons ground cinnamon
- 1 cup quick oats
- 1 teaspoon dried ginger
- ¾ cup butter

Method:

1. Stir all the ingredients in the crockpot.
2. Cook on high for 1 hour.

Nutritional Value:

- Calories 387
- Total Fat 24.4g
- Saturated Fat 14.8g
- Cholesterol 61mg
- Sodium 167mg
- Total Carbohydrate 43.6g
- Dietary Fiber 8.5g
- Total Sugars 24.1g
- Protein 2.7g
- Potassium 339mg

Conclusion

With the help of this book, you can now start your journey to weight loss and better health.

This book provides you with countless delicious and healthy recipes that can be prepared without the stress and hassle using the ever-reliable crockpot.

So are you ready to get started? Good luck!